The Diabetes Solution

Take Control of Your Blood Sugar & Restore Your Health Naturally

Christine Weil

Christine Weil

© 2014

Disclaimer and Terms of Use: The Author and Publisher have strived to be as accurate and complete as possible in the creation of this book, notwithstanding the fact that they do not warrant or represent at any time that the contents within are accurate due to the rapidly changing nature of the Internet. While all attempts have been made to verify information provided in this publication, the Author and Publisher assume no responsibility for errors, omissions, or contrary interpretation of the subject matter herein. Any perceived slights of specific persons, peoples, or organizations are unintentional. In practical advice books, like anything else in life, there are no guarantees of income made or health benefits received. This book is not intended for use as a source of medical, legal, business, accounting or financial advice. All readers are advised to seek services of competent professionals in medical, legal, business, accounting, and finance matters.

Printed in the United States of America

Table of Contents

Introduction

Congratulations on deciding to take control of your Type II Diabetes. Purchasing your copy of *The Diabetes Solution: Take Control of Your Blood Sugar & Restore Your Health Naturally* is the first step in beginning your journey to a healthier you!

Chances are that if you are reading this guide, either you or a loved one is suffering from the symptoms associated with Type II Diabetes. The information provided here will explain what Type II Diabetes is, associated symptoms, and effective treatments. It will also provide you with guidance about lifestyle choices, portion control, and how to shop for healthy foods. Finally, there are some recipes for you to try which are specifically designed for Type II Diabetics and are quite delicious!

After finishing this guide, you should be well equipped both emotionally and physically for the changes you need to make to take control of your blood sugar.

While you are working on controlling your blood sugar, keep this guide handy for guidance, recipes, and tips for maintaining a normal levels and encouragement.

We know there are a lot of options out there concerning Diabetes, so Thank You for choosing *The Diabetes Solution*.

I hope you enjoy it!

Christine Weil

What is Type II Diabetes?

Type II Diabetes - also known as non-insulin dependent Diabetes Mellitus - is a chronic metabolic disorder that can occur for a multitude of reasons. Symptoms include muscle pain, excessive thirst, fatigue, and excessive urination. It is an extremely common chronic disorder, but unlike many medical conditions it can be reversed with proper diet, exercise, and an overall active lifestyle.

Considered an epidemic by the World Health Organization, 314 million people worldwide suffer from this chronic disease. This type of Diabetes is typically seen in adults who are overweight or obese due to lifestyle choices, though research indicates that up to 5% of sufferers have an inherited genetic disorder.

An insidious disease, Type II Diabetes develops slowly over time and often remains undiagnosed until a health crisis or a routine health exam reveals an elevated fasting blood sugar. The diagnosis of Type II Diabetes has increased rapidly since the 1980's and continues to rise every year. In fact, 30% of Americans currently have Type II Diabetes and this number will increase to 50% by 2020. If incident rates continue to increase as projected by the World health Organization, Type II Diabetes will be the 7th leading cause of death worldwide by 2030. With these kinds of numbers, chances are that either you or a loved one is affected. Fortunately, this book contains valuable information which could help to prevent further symptoms or reverse Type II Diabetes completely!

Though this information seems a little scary and maybe overwhelming, you have already taken the first step by purchasing this book. Designed to help you take charge of your health and life, we will discuss the symptoms, susceptible individuals, and then provide you with lifestyle tips that are easy to follow. We believe that everyone deserves to live a long, healthy, and fulfilling life. The methods described in this book will change your life if you are ready to learn and put in the hard work. So now that you're ready, let's get started!

Symptoms

The symptoms associated with Type II Diabetes are varied and can be confused with symptoms of many other disease processes, but typically the following are indicators that you or a loved one may be suffering from this condition:

- Polydipsia – excessive thirst
- Muscle pain
- Frequent and long lasting infections
- Polyuria – excessive urination
- Fatigue
- Hunger
- Blurry vision or other vision changes
- Neuropathy – unexplained localized or systemic pain

Less Common Symptoms

- Ketoacidosis: Increase in blood pH due to an error in lipid metabolism
- Microalbuminuria: Albumin in the urine
- Glucosuria: Glucose in the urine
- Proteinuria: Protein in the urine
- Loss of feeling in limbs
- Urinary tract infections
- Gangrene resulting from unnoticed injuries and infections

Though these are common symptoms, they are also present in a variety of other disorders. For example, Hyponatremia, Schizophrenia, and Diabtes Insipidus are all diseases which cause polydipsia and polyuria. Glomerulonephritis – a kidney disorder – can cause microalbuminuria and proteinuria. Therefore it is important to rule out other chronic diseases by getting a physical examination and laboratory testing from a physician or naturopath. If no other disease process is seen, Type II Diabetes should be suspected.

Some of the less common symptoms are extremely dangerous to your health. Normal urine output should contain nothing but sterile urine and excess electrolytes. When compounds such as glucose, albumin, and protein are found in the urine it is an indicator that the kidneys are permanently damaged.

Going forward, it is important that you understand that it is up to you protect your health. Only you can decide that today is the day that you begin to live your life in a healthy and active way. You will need to commit to following the guidelines of this book as well as recommendations by your physician.

With exercise, a low-calorie/high nutrition diet, and a combination of pharmaceuticals and natural remedies, I know that you can achieve your goal of controlling your Diabetes and living a long healthy life.

As a precaution, you should know that this information is not intended to replace the advice of a licensed and highly educated professional; it is meant to lead you in the right direction for a healthier life. Please discuss any health concerns with your doctor, as this book is not intended for diagnostic purposes.

So now that you understand exactly what Type II Diabetes is, let's take a look at the basic physiology behind blood sugar regulation and discuss the major causes.

What Are The Causes?

To understand how Type II Diabetes develops, it is important to first understand the basic anatomy and physiology associated with the pancreas. The pancreas is a gland located in the abdomen behind the stomach and is part of the endocrine system. With many important functions, the pancreas secretes hormones like insulin and glucagon. Though both are vital to blood sugar regulation, insulin is the hormone which does not function properly in Type II Diabetes. This improper function is known as insulin resistance, which we will explore further later in this chapter. First, let's take a look at how insulin is produced.

Insulin is secreted by cells within the pancreas known as beta islet cells. In Type I Diabetes, these cells are destroyed either through an auto-immune response or due to infection. In Type II Diabetes, these cells remain intact; it is a combination of improper insulin secretion and dysfunctional muscle, liver, and fat cells that cause problems in blood sugar regulation.

The functionality of insulin and muscle, liver, and fat cells varies within the diabetic population. For some, insulin is secreted normally and it is other cells involved in blood sugar regulation which are dysfunctional. For others, the beta islet cells do not secrete insulin properly though damage is not present and the liver, muscle, and fat cells function normally. In many instances, it is a combination of these two processes which lead to insulin resistance and Type II Diabetes.

It is important to note that insulin resistance is not quite the same as Type II Diabetes; they are two distinct chronic diseases related to one another. A person may have insulin resistance but not Type II Diabetes. You can think of insulin resistance as a precursor to Type II Diabetes as the symptoms are less severe and without proper lifestyle changes will lead to Type II Diabetes.

Fortunately, most cases of Type II Diabetes and insulin resistance can be reversed completely by significant changes to diet and lifestyle, especially when combined with the naturopathic techniques found in this book. If you put in the time and effort and commit to significant lifestyle changes, you can be free of this chronic disease. It may take some time to see the effects of these lifestyle changes, but stick with the program and you will be amazed when you finally do!

Who is Most Likely To Have Type II Diabetes?

Though Diabetes can strike almost anyone especially if someone is genetically at risk, the following groups are the most likely to acquire Type II Diabetes:

- Overweight or obese individuals
- American Indians
- Black Americans
- Pacific Islanders
- Women
- Anyone older than 45 years of age
- Asian Americans
- Hispanic or Latino Americans

If this seems like a large proportion of Americans, it is! More than two-thirds of Americans fit into these groups. Additionally, one of the fastest growing groups of Type II Diabetics is children. Children as young as 8 years old are being diagnosed with obesity related Diabetes, high blood pressure, and high cholesterol due to lack of exercise and poor diet choices.

It is important to note that diet and inactivity are chiefly to blame for the 30% of individuals suffering from Type II Diabetes. As Americans, we all love rich, salty foods as well as decadent sweets (I'm guilty too). In many ways, the majority of us are addicted to salt, sugar, and the other synthetic compounds found in our favorite foods. We all know that is bad for our health, but it can be hard to resist with all the rushing around we do. It is often more convenient to grab something quick and eat on the way to wherever we are going. And at the end of the day, it feels great to kick up your feet and watch the boob tube even when a walk would be just as relaxing.

For these reasons, as well as a personal desire to look and feel better, it is so important to embrace a healthy lifestyle today. By eating the right foods in the right proportions and exercising at least three times per week, not only will you look better, but you will feel amazing!

Now that you know who is at risk, we can talk about how Type II Diabetes is diagnosed by a physician or naturopath. Though it can be daunting to visit a doctor's office, we have provided all the information you need to feel comfortable and get the most from your visit in the very next chapter!

Diagnostics

Type II Diabetes is undiagnosed for a majority of individuals and is only discovered through an emergency or through a routine physical exam. So, the first step in being diagnosed is to schedule a physical exam with a licensed physician or naturopath. Once you have kept your appointment, your physician will do a physical exam looking for indicators of disease. Some symptoms of Type II Diabetes are apparent in your skin, eyes, and body fat distribution.

For example, an undiagnosed Diabetic may have acne, scaly skin, and unexplained rashes. Affected individuals may also have infections in the folds of their skin as well as their armpits and groin area. This is because bacteria and yeast LOVE sugars and Type II Diabetics typically have plenty to go around. Also present is discoloration of the skin around the nose, chin, and neck which makes these areas appear rougher and darker than other parts of your body.

Another common finding upon examination is the presence of excess fat in the abdominal region. This excess fat directly contributes to Type II Diabetes as well as a variety of other chronic diseases including heart disease and hormonal disorders.

After the physical exam, your doctor will probably order a panel of tests including a complete metabolic panel (CMP), a glycated hemoglobin (A1C), and an analysis of your urine (UA). It is these tests that will provide definitive proof that you are or are not suffering from Type II Diabetes.

The CMP evaluates your kidney and liver functions as well a blood pH and the level of sugar present in your blood. The A1C provides information about your blood sugar levels over the last three months. The UA looks at what is in your urine, which shouldn't be much. You will probably have these tests every few months if you do have any symptoms of Diabetes

If you have Type II Diabetes the CMP will reveal high blood sugar levels and depending on how long you have been undiagnosed, abnormal kidney and liver function as well as an abnormal blood pH. The UA will reveal protein and sugar in your urine, which also indicates kidney damage.

At first this might not make sense as these tests don't really have anything to with your pancreas, which we have already blamed for Diabetes. Though it's a little confusing, when your blood sugar is high and insulin is not doing its job, your body begins looking for other ways to eliminate the excess sugar. The kidneys and liver act as filters and anytime we have excess amounts of blood based nutrients or compounds, these organs go to work getting rid of them. These organs are not built to process such large molecules as proteins and sugars and as a result they take a beating.

However, these findings do not necessarily mean that you will forever have kidney and liver problems, it just means that it is time to make some lifestyle changes. Your physician will (or already has) provided information related to diet, exercise, and synthetic medications. From here it is up to you educate yourself further and decide your next step.

In the end, the responsibility of getting well is up to you. Physicians can provide plenty of information and guidance, but ultimately you have to decide what kind of life you want to lead. It is also up to you to decide if you want to take synthetic pharmaceuticals or more natural treatments to regulate your blood sugar. Only you can decide what kind of diet and exercise will benefit you the most in the long run. Fortunately, by purchasing this guide you are already well are your way to attaining your goals of being happy and healthy.

All it takes now is commitment to yourself, your family, and change.

Armed with all of this information, you should now be ready to look at treatment options, both synthetic and natural. With the help of this guide and your physician, you can make decisions that will change your life for the better. Are you ready to start?

Western/Pharmaceutical Medications

Western medicine typically relies heavily on synthetic medications produced by pharmaceutical companies to regulate their patients' blood sugars. A few popular examples of prescribed medications are:

- Metformin
- Glipizide
- Januvia

However, recent research indicates that these medications are not particularly good for blood sugar regulation; especially Metformin. Additionally, the above listed medications can have severe side effects including multisystem organ failure.

So why do physicians keep prescribing them? The answer is because that is what they are trained to do; see a problem, treat it with meds. Many physicians that practice western medicine only see the diagnosis and often do not take the time to see the whole person.

As lifestyle choices such as stress, poor diet, lack of sleep, and inactivity all contribute to Type II Diabetes, it is important to look at an individual's entire life. This is not to say that pharmaceuticals don't work for some people or that western medicine doesn't care about your life, it is just to point out that other options are available for your complete care.

In the next section we will discuss alternatives to the traditional pharmaceutical approach to controlling Type II Diabetes. Many options are available and most likely a combination of traditional and alternative approaches will be the ticket to regulating your blood sugar.

Natural Treatments

Diabetes is a disease that has existed at least as long as history has been recorded. Before the late 1800's very little pharmaceutical intervention existed and humans relied on natural remedies to control Diabetes and its varied symptoms. The following are some excellent alternatives to western medications.

Blood Sugar Regulators

Biotin – Biotin is a vitamin which increases the activation of glucokinase, the first enzyme in the metabolism process of glucose in the liver. Glucokinase in Diabetics tends to be lower than those who do not have Diabetes which leads to trouble regulating blood sugars. By increasing the blood glucokinase levels, insulin sensitivity is improved.

Dehydroepiandrosterone – DHEA is an adrenal hormone which is proven to help with blood sugar regulation. Scientists don't know exactly why DHEA is so useful, but leading research indicates that it boosts glucose metabolism within the liver. It also helps to improve beta cell function which reduces insulin resistance and it helps obese patients to lose weight.

Chromium and Magnesium – These trace minerals are an important supplements for Type II Diabetes because they improve the breakdown of proteins, carbohydrates, and fats. By aiding in metabolism, Chromium and Magnesium help to control blood sugar levels. Recent human clinical trials indicate that when taken in conjunction with Indian Gooseberry, fasting blood sugars were reduced by fifteen percent after two months of therapy.

Cinnamon – This common spice has been used for centuries in Ayurvedic and Greco-Roman medicine. With a lot of medicinal properties, it is especially good at stabilizing blood sugars as well as increasing insulin sensitivity. It is important to note that cinnamon in its household form is not the same as the medicinal form. For medical benefits to be seen a water soluble extract must be used.

Tianqi – A traditional mix of ten Chinese herbs, Tianqi is taken in a capsule. It has been proven in multiple clinical trials to prevent pre-diabetes from developing into Type II Diabetes. It also has been proven to be just as effective as Metformin, a popular synthetic medication. Made to the specifications of the Chinese version of the FDA, this capsule should be relatively free of contaminants.

Pain and Damage Reducers

Alpha Lipoic Acid – ALA is an anti-oxidant which can help to relieve nerve pain, burning sensations, and numbness. It can also be used to improve diabetes related vision issues and helps to reverse cardiac damage. ALA also naturally breaks down carbohydrates, which provides much needed energy to your organs.

Vitamin E – Vitamin E is one of the most effective natural therapies available today. Not only does it decrease the risk of actually acquiring Type II Diabetes, it also helps to heal damage caused by uncontrolled Diabetes. For example, taking Vitamin E can help with diabetic neuropathy, cardiac damage, as well as prevent cataracts; all very common symptoms of uncontrolled Diabetes. Like many other natural treatments, Vitamin E also improves insulin sensitivity leading to better controlled blood sugar levels.

N-acetyl-L-cysteine – NAC is an antioxidant commonly used to treat overdoses of acetaminophen. This is not its only use however. Recent studies suggest that taken with Vitamin E, NAC can help to control heart damage in Diabetics and is perhaps even capable of preventing heart attacks.

Garlic – A super supplement, the active compound in garlic is Allium. Allium aids in glutathione production which in turn does quite a lot for the health of any individual. It helps to prevent cardiac damage, promotes weight loss, increases insulin sensitivity, lowers blood pressure, and lowers cholesterol. All of these benefits are particularly important for a Diabetic as many eventually suffer from cardiac disease, high blood pressure, and high cholesterol. If you choose to use any supplements choose this one!

Quercetin – Considered a flavinoid, quercetin is an antioxidant that also stabilizes levels of essential vitamins and minerals. Capable of reducing blood pressure by relieving Diabetes associated inflammation in the vascular system. Quercetin does not help to regulate blood sugars or improve insulin sensitivity so it should be taken with another natural remedy or a pharmaceutical such as Metformin. It is most effective at lower doses of around 500 mg.

Omega 3 Fatty acids and Omega 6 Fatty Acids – Considered essential for optimal health, omega fatty acids can help in a variety of ways. Omega 3 is found in fish oil and significantly decreases inflammation associated with Type II Diabetes which prevents heart disease in some cases. Omega 6 is present in the supplement GLA and helps with diabetic neuropathy. However, it must be taken regularly and for at least a year for all the benefits to be seen.

Lifestyle Changes and Non-Medicinal Treatments

Moving forward in this guide we will be focusing on lifestyle changes instead of medications. You will see information about why you may be overindulging in certain foods, how you can identify the problem, and ways to change your behavior. Then you will see information about food choices, some general guidelines regarding grocery shopping, and some great recipes. Lastly, we will discuss becoming more active so that you can lose weight and keep your Diabetes under control.

In addition to natural and synthetic medications, it will also take a significant commitment to weight loss, exercise, and a healthy low calorie diet in order to control your blood sugar. To be successful, you will have to admit to yourself, your physicians, and your family that you have an issue with diet and exercise. For only you can decide to change your life for the better!

Before beginning a diet and exercise program, record your current eating habits, daily activities, and daily moods for two weeks. This will help you to see exactly which habits need to be changed in order to be successful. It will also help you understand what your motivations are when you overindulge or fail to exercise. Perhaps something went wrong during your day so you grabbed a candy bar. Or perhaps your significant other is already sitting on the couch enjoying a soda when you get home, so you skip your planned walk. Whatever the reasons, you have to understand and accept your flaws before you can move on.

For some, it may help to try **Cognitive Behavioral Therapy** (also known as talk therapy) to correct bad habits and help you to deal with your impulses. During this kind of therapy you will work to identify negative behavioral patterns preventing you from achieving your goals. Once a behavioral pattern is identified, various coping mechanisms can be used to defeat these behaviors.

For example, let's say it is your habit to eat a candy bar on the way home as you wind down from work, even if you aren't hungry. This could be an indicator that you are eating for emotional comfort which is a very poor coping mechanism as it is harmful to your health. A better coping mechanism would be listening to music or an audiobook to relieve stress. Or if you like learning new things, NPR offers many free podcasts on many interesting topics. If your mind is engaged in learning, you won't be looking to food for stress relief.

Another good example could be stopping at the gas station in the morning to get a large coffee or soda even if you don't feel tired. It could be that is a morning ritual or a way of soothing anxiety during a long commute. A better coping mechanism would be to brew a cup of green tea if you need something to sip on. Green tea is rich with antioxidants and has less caffeine than a cup of coffee. It also helps to regulate blood sugar levels and creates a sense of satiety (fullness).

Gaining positive coping mechanisms can be accomplished with the help of a Cognitive Behavioral Therapy workbook or with a licensed clinical therapist. As long as you are doing the work to eliminate behaviors that stand in the way of your goals, it doesn't really matter whether you work on your own or with a therapist. The important thing is that you find a way to live a healthy and fulfilled life. If you are having trouble improving on your own though, you should visit your physician or make an appointment with a therapist. There is absolutely nothing wrong with reaching out for help when you need it, especially when it concerns your emotional and physical health.

Non-Medicinal Treatments

In addition to diet/exercise modification and creating positive coping mechanisms, you can try other activities such as lymphatic massage, meditation, acupuncture, and herbal body wraps. If this sounds like a day at the spa, you are right! What we consider today to be indulgences others have been using for centuries as medical treatment. In fact, in Europe and Asia medical massage, acupuncture, meditation, and herbal body wraps are prescribed by both physicians and naturopaths for a variety of health issues including Diabetes. To better understand why these "spa" practices are actually medical treatments, we will now spend some time discussing each method in terms of physiology.

Medical lymphatic message is a message therapy which specifically focuses on eliminating excess body fluid, relieving inflammation, and ridding your body of toxins. This is accomplished by encouraging your lymph system to drain excess fluids from your body therefore preventing the painful swelling in extremities commonly associate with obesity and Type II Diabetes. Typically this is accomplished by applying a specific amount of continuous pressure in a circular motion to the swollen areas or lymph nodes. A naturopath can teach you to do this at home or can recommend a professional to do it for you, but either way the result is the same; your lymphatic system is stimulated to remove excess fluid and toxins which may be affecting your health.

Acupuncture is another method of removing toxins from your body and increasing circulation. At first glance it may seem a little scary to you and that is ok, but acupuncture is widely recognized as an effective treatment for many medical conditions including Diabetes. A certified acupuncturist knows exactly which areas to stimulate in order to relieve stress, decrease pain, remove toxins, and improve circulation; all extremely important to staying healthy as a Type II Diabetic. Though it should be easy to locate an acupuncturist, you may feel better if your naturopath or physician recommends a certified professional so that you feel safe and comfortable with your treatments.

Herbal body wraps are not only pleasurable, but with the right combination of herbs and heat it can be an extremely effective way of removing toxins and excess fluids as well as improving circulation. Done properly, the process involves being wrapped inside multiple layers of different fabrics drenched in beneficial herbs.

After about 40 minutes of intense heat, your body should have rid itself of toxins and excess fluids. Because of the heat requirements, it is important to come to your appointment well hydrated and to continue drinking cold water during treatment. This prevents dehydration as well as overheating. The point is not to sweat out all the extra water in your body, but encourage the lymphatic system to drain fluid and to improve the vascular system. Both of these integral systems are negatively affected by Type II Diabetes and without intervention can lead to significant heart issues.

Meditation is an effective way to not only relieve stress, but to gain focus and perspective on your goals. It has been used across all cultures for thousands of years. The meaning of meditation is different for everyone, but there are basics which apply to anyone engaging in meditation.

To begin you must find a quiet spot free from distractions and clear your mind of all thoughts. For beginners, it sometimes helps to breathe in for eight seconds, hold for two seconds, and breathe out for eight seconds. Concentrating on your breathing gives you a focal point allowing you to relax deeply and escape from the world briefly. Research has proven that engaging in daily meditation for as few as fifteen minutes results in decreased anxiety, depression, blood pressure, and negativity. Overall people that meditate are healthier, deal with stress better, and experience a higher quality of living than those that don't.

If you find it hard to keep thoughts from interrupting your meditation time just by breathing, try using a positive phrase or mantra to keep you focused. For example, it may help for you to repeat a calming or inspiration religious quote instead of counting your breaths. You could also try envisioning an especially relaxing place including the way it smells, sounds, and feels.

For some, unguided meditation does not work. Fortunately, there are many forms of meditation including yoga and worship services. If these aren't options for you, you may want to contact a therapist or hypnotist as they can guide you into a meditative state with specialized techniques, a safe environment, and a soothing voice. In time you may be able to replicate this at home or during exercise for additional stress release.

However you get there, the point of a meditative state is to release tension and negativity by focusing on something outside of the normal day to day. By not allowing thoughts to race through your head, you may find that you are able to gain perspective on what is keeping you from achieving your goals. You also may find that it gives you the inner peace and strength to handle stress without contributing to your Diabetic symptoms. As Diabetics often have heart disease, it is important not to allow stress to creep in.

In an above paragraph I mentioned a hypnotist. Many people regard hypnotism as a party trick or do not believe in it all, but it has been researched by healthcare professionals and there is something to it.

A trained hypnotist can help you to stop smoking, banish negative thoughts, and change the way you feel about food and exercise. If you are really struggling to change your habits and have tried other methods without success, it may be a good idea to make an appointment with a therapist that practices hypnotherapy. He/she may be able to train your subconscious to think differently ultimately leading to your success in your goals! When it comes to your health, it is sometimes necessary to try things that you previously had not considered. For those with Type II Diabetes, for which there is no medical cure, it especially important to find something that works for you.

I know all of this information is a lot to consider, but you don't have to do it all by yourself. You aren't alone in your journey towards better health as this guide will next explore recipes, exercises, and give you online resources for finding a physician, naturopath, or therapist to help you get where you to be!

The next few sections will help you to better understand how to prepare your meals, how much to eat, which foods to avoid, and how to exercise so that you can get more out of life. These methods are completely natural and are scientifically proven to help you control your blood sugar levels and feel great without synthetic medication. It helps that our sample diet plan and exercises are easy and fun!

Calorie Recommendations, Portion Control, and Grocery Shopping

Now that you know that accountability and healthy coping mechanisms are essential to achieving your health goals, let's explore calories, portion control, and grocery shopping. In addition to medication and supplements, eating the right foods in the right amount will help you to lose weight and stabilize your blood sugar. As most Type II Diabetes cases are completely reversible with diet and exercise, it is one of the most, if not the most important components of controlling your blood sugar levels and overall health.

A good mantra to have as you move forward is that calories in must be equal to calories out in order to maintain your weight. If you are looking to lose weight, then you must expend more calories than you are eating. If it sounds simple, it's because the concept is simple. It is the self-control part of the equation that is so difficult especially if you are used to eating too many processed foods whenever you want.

For a non-overweight moderately active individual 2000 calories for women, and 2600 calories for men, is sufficient for all your nutritional needs. Of course this varies slightly by age and activity level, but typically no more than the noted calories should be consumed in one day. For someone who is overweight and who does not engage in exercise, this calorie requirement is significantly lower. Statistics support this and as you will see, it is disturbing how few people actually fall into the "active" 2000 calories a day group.

Less than twenty-five percent of Americans participate in any activity other than the walking required to participate in life. This means that other than walking around at work or the grocery store or walking to and from their cars, seventy-five percent of adults do not engage in any other physical activity. As current recommendations state that adults need to engage in at least 150 minutes of moderate activity and weight training per week, it is clear that most of us fall into the seventy-five percent; including you. It is also clear that for most us, 2000 calories a day is too many.

Remedying the discrepancy between your activity level versus the amount of calories you consume is easier than you may think. With tools like myplate.gov and other government supported organizations, understanding your lifestyle is easier than ever. You can enter each food item you consume and applications like MyPlate will calculate the calorie amount and will also tally the nutritional value of that item.

At the end of the day, you will have the amount of calories you have eaten as well as your nutritional status. If you have not met your daily fruit and vegetable requirement or you are deficient in a certain vitamin or mineral, MyPlate will give your this information. It makes being accountable and staying on track as easy as recording your status on Facebook!

Once you know what you are doing right and what you are doing wrong nutritionally, you can change your shopping habits to get the most out of your diet program. For the most part, this will mean eliminating most processed foods, junk foods, and simple carbohydrates like white bread. Frozen items should also be avoided unless they are organic and full of lean protein like chicken or fish, vegetables, and complex carbohydrates like brown rice or quinoa. Look for items that are low in sodium and sugar, but high in fiber and vitamins. This can easily be accomplished by doing what is called "shopping the perimeter".

Shopping the perimeter means avoiding the middle isles of a grocery store where most of the processed foods live. It means sticking to the produce, dairy, and meat sections.

Choosing fresh fruits and vegetables along with lean meats and low fat dairy items will ensure that you are getting all the nutrition and energy you need for as little calories as possible.

This concept of a low calorie diet might be confusing because in the beginning you will not feel full and you will crave your favorite junk foods. The word "starving" may constantly enter your thoughts. Fortunately, changing the way you think about the purpose of eating will help you to resist this temptation and eventually be fulfilled by a healthy diet.

Food is now and always has been fuel for our bodies. It might help for you to think about your body as a gas tank. When you go to the station to fill up the gas tank, you know that only a certain amount of gas will fit. Externally, you can hear the click of the pump when the tank is full. If that mechanism is broken, the gas tank will overflow because it cannot accept any more fuel. Your body is the same way, but instead of hearing an external click you might hear the grumblings of indigestion.

After eating too much, your body also "overflows" in a sense. If you overfill your stomach, it begins a process called "dumping". Normally your stomach does a good deal of the digestion process, churning food for about 2-3 hours in a chemical mixture that breaks down your food in preparation for your intestines. When you overeat, your stomach becomes too full to digest and "dumps" the contents of your stomach into your intestines regardless of whether or not the food is digested enough.

Overfilling your gas tank can result in many health problems, but for a Type II Diabetic specifically it can wreak havoc on your blood sugar levels. Constantly having high blood sugar can cause you to be drowsy, irritable, and fatigued. It also contributes to heart, liver, kidney, and eye disease, ultimately leading to a shorter life expectancy.

The diet, exercise, and emotional changes in this chapter can be challenging. Perhaps it is the biggest challenge you have encountered so far in your life, but it is the most worthwhile to face. When your health begins to improve and you start seeing the results of all of your hard work and dedication, I promise you will be glad you did it; so will your family and friends.

The Importance of Celebrating Milestones

When you are working hard to achieve your health goals, it can be easy to fall into melancholy and can decrease your drive. As this contributes to weight gain, it is important to create milestones during your journey. Milestones and rewards give you a clear direction, even more motivation, and a sense of accomplishment. Celebrating is important to your continued success and will push you forward when you feel like giving up. The reward shouldn't be food related, but should make you feel good about your progress and be something you really want.

For example, if you plan to lose thirty pounds in two months also plan a reward. For some people that is a material reward like a few new wardrobe items in your new size. For others it is a break from all the hard work in the form of a trip or a "staycation". Whatever you choose, involve your family and friends.

If you are the family or friend of someone suffering from Diabetes, cheer on your loved one! You are their motivation for getting their blood sugar under control and your support can mean the difference in whether they are successful or not.

Praise is a powerful tool, so use it often when your loved one follows through. Even if the milestone seems small to you, be lavish in your praise; it is not a small milestone for your family member or friend. Be encouraging and if you can, offer your support as they change their life for the better. If this isn't something you excel at or if you tend to be negative, try your very best to offer support.

If you are a family member, you may be feeling a little out of sorts yourself during this transition. Being a caregiver or someone to lean on when times are hard can be stressful too. Be sure to take care of yourself as well and seek advice from a therapist or physician if you need it. Being someone's support system is not meant to be at your expense, so please don't let it be.

Failures and Forgiveness

As someone working hard to achieve goals that may seem impossible, it is important to recognize that you may fail periodically, in fact you *probably will* at times, and that's OK!

Failure is a normal part of everyone's life and should be taken in stride. This is not your high school science class, or college health class where failure is a "catastrophic event," failure here is a learning experience and an opportunity to practice a little self-love. Do not waste your time feeling lousy about not achieving an established goal; learn from it and move on!

Look at your mistakes objectively and without blame. If you know you were snacking when you shouldn't have been, use the disappointment of your failure as motivation to succeed next time. Do not wallow in self-pity, make excuses, or play the part of a victim. Own your life and your actions, the good *and* the bad. Be willing to allow yourself to grow as an individual for your health's sake.

Remember that becoming a new person takes time; you won't become the healthy individual you want to be overnight! Change is inherently challenging and time consuming. No one can be expected to be perfect on the very first attempt. Decide that your need to be healthy is a journey and a long one at that. Be disciplined, but stay positive too. There is no benefit from beating yourself up, only more problems.

As Eleanor Roosevelt so wisely said "You gain strength, courage, and confidence by every experience in which you really stop to look fear in the face. You are able to say to yourself…I lived through this horror. I can take the next thing that comes along."

Healthy and Delicious Recipes

Since most people love eating (I know I do!), this part should be especially fun to explore. The recipes featured here are not only good for controlling your blood sugar, but they are also low in fat and calories while being rich in nutrients. As you learn more about eating healthy, you will discover that healthy food is not necessarily bland food and your body will begin to actually crave the healthy foods.

Using various spices, citrus, and vinegars can make almost any meal seem like it is straight from a restaurant. In fact, many chefs use these ingredients to make their dishes shine! Adding just a hint of spice or bitterness is the key to making a delicious and low calorie meal.

I have provided a few recipes; I hope that you enjoy each and every one. I also hope that it will motivate you to learn more healthy recipes that fuel your body and your journey towards being disease free!

*All recipes are courtesy of Januvia. More can be found at:

http://www.januvia.com/sitagliptin/januvia/consumer/living-with-diabetes/healthy-eating/healthy-recipes/breakfast/index.jsp

Nicoise Salad

Prep Time: 10
minutes
Total Time: 10
minutes
Serves: 4

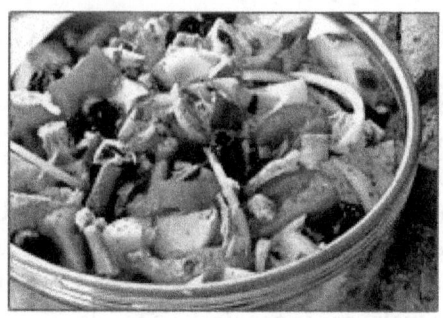

Ingredients

6 cups ready-to-serve romaine lettuce
6 ounces canned albacore tuna in water, drained
2 baked potatoes, unpeeled, sliced
2 cups cooked green beans
8 black pitted olives
2 ripe plum tomatoes, sliced
¼ cup balsamic vinegar
¼ teaspoon black pepper

Preparation:

1. Place lettuce in a large salad bowl.
2. Top with tuna, sliced potatoes, green beans, olives, and tomatoes.
3. Cover and refrigerate until ready to serve.
4. Serve salad with balsamic vinegar and black pepper on top.

Make-Ahead Tossed Salad

Prep Time: 5 minutes or less
Total Time: 5 minutes or less
Serves: 10

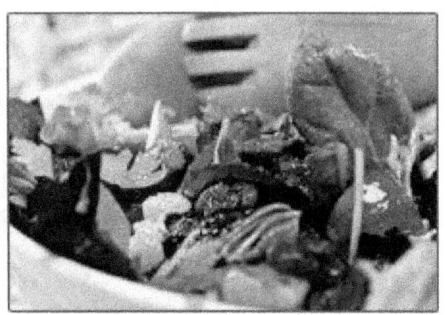

Ingredients

10 cups romaine lettuce (1 head), chopped
5 cups cabbage, shredded (½ head)
2 cups grated carrots (2 carrots)
Optional toppings: Dried herbs, tomatoes, cucumbers, onions, nuts.

Preparation:

1. Wash romaine under cold running water and allow to drain in colander.
2. Add cabbage and carrots plus any of the optional toppings you're planning to use.
3. Place all in large bag and refrigerate until ready to use, up to 3 days.
4. Serve with flavored vinegar or nonfat salad dressing.

Tortilla Pizza

Prep Time: 5 minutes or less
Total Time: 5 minutes or less
Serves: 1

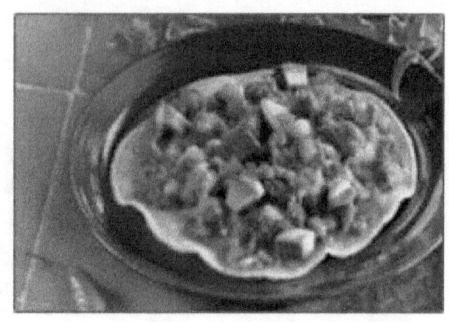

Ingredients

1 whole-wheat flour tortilla
1/4 cup broccoli florets, chopped
1/4 cup green onions, chopped
1/4 cup mushrooms, sliced
1/4 cup no salt added tomato sauce
1/4 cup reduced-fat shredded cheese
1/4 teaspoon dried oregano

Preparation:

1. Preheat oven to 400°F.
2. Place tortilla on a cookie tray.
3. Top with the sauce, broccoli, onions, and mushrooms.
4. Sprinkle with cheese and oregano.
5. Bake the pizza until the cheese is melted, about 5 minutes.
6. Cut in 4 and serve hot.

We recommend serving this pizza with a large green salad.

Mile-High Veggie Burger

Prep Time: 10 minutes
Total Time: 15 minutes or less
Serves: 4

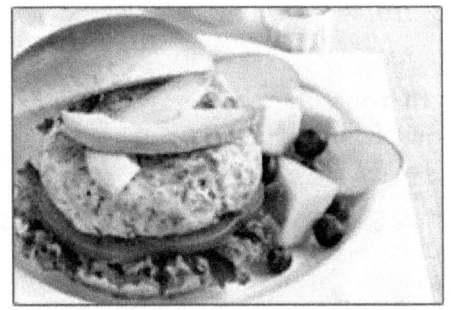

Ingredients

- 4 vegetarian burger patties
- 4 whole-grain rolls
- 2 cups dark green lettuce, shredded
- 2 tomatoes, sliced
- 1/2 cup sliced red onion
- 4 tablespoons no-sugar-added ketchup

Preparation:

1. Heat vegetarian burgers in your microwave or toaster oven until thoroughly heated, about 1 minute per patty.
2. Toast the rolls, if desired. Split the rolls and place the burger on the bottom half.
3. Top each burger with 1/2 cup lettuce, 2 or 3 slices of tomato, 2 slices of red onion, and 1 tablespoon of ketchup.
4. Serve immediately.

Serving suggestion: We like to serve this burger with fresh-cut veggie sticks and low-fat coleslaw.

Halibut with Teriyaki Sauce

Prep Time: 10 minutes
Total Time: 10 minutes
Serves: 4

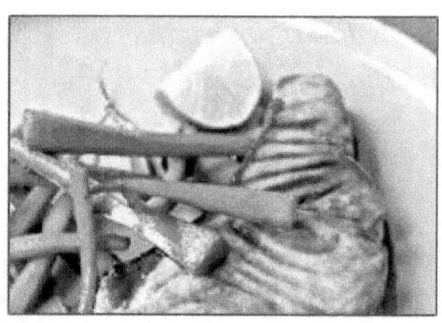

Ingredients

4 fluid ounces pineapple juice
3 tablespoons teriyaki sauce, no sugar added
1 tablespoon reduced-calorie pancake syrup
¾ teaspoon cornstarch
¼ teaspoon garlic powder
1/8 teaspoon cayenne pepper, ground
1 ½ pounds halibut
2 tablespoons bread crumbs, seasoned
1 tablespoon canola oil

Preparation:

1. Combine pineapple juice, teriyaki sauce, syrup, cornstarch, garlic powder and cayenne in a small bowl.
2. Stir well with a whisk and set aside.
3. Rinse fish; pat dry with paper towels.
4. Cut fish into six 6-ounce pieces, if necessary.
5. Place fish in a large, plastic resealable food storage bag along with bread crumbs. Seal and shake to coat; set aside.
6. Spread black pepper on a large plate. Remove fish, reserving marinade and onion. Press both sides into pepper to coat and set aside.
7. Heat oil in a large non-stick skillet over medium heat.

8. Add fish and cook 4 minutes on each side or until fish flakes easily with a fork.
9. Remove fish from skillet; set aside, and keep warm.
10. Add teriyaki mixture to skillet.
11. Bring to a boil. Cook for 1 minute, stirring constantly.
12. Spoon over fish to serve.

Crunchy Lemon Parmesan Fish

Prep Time: 15 minutes
Total Time: 20 minutes
Serves: 4

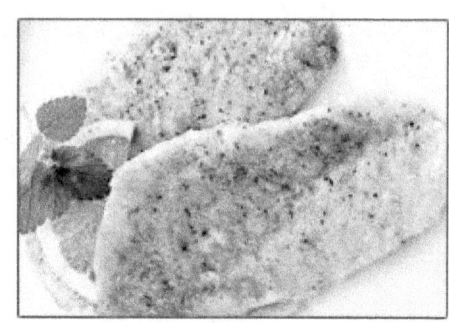

Ingredients

1 pound sole/flounder, uncooked
1 cup cereal, whole-grain fortified flakes
1 tablespoon Parmesan cheese, fat free
1 tablespoon butter
1 teaspoon lemon peel
1/4 teaspoon black pepper

Preparation:

1. Preheat oven to 450°F.
2. Rinse fish; pat dry with paper towels. Cut into four 4-ounce portions, if necessary.
3. Lightly coat a jelly-roll pan or other shallow baking pan with olive oil. Place fish in prepared pan, tucking under any thin edges so you have an even thickness.
4. Crush cereal into coarse crumbs (a couple spins in the food processor is great for this).
5. In a small bowl, combine crushed cereal, Parmesan cheese, butter (melted), lemon peel (grated or shredded), and pepper.
6. Sprinkle crumb mixture on top of fish. Bake for 4 to 6 minutes per 1/2-inch thickness of fish or until fish flakes easily with a fork and crumbs are brown.
7. Serve with lemon wedges, if desired.

Cincinnati Chili

Prep Time: 15
minutes
Total Time: 70
minutes
Serves: 4

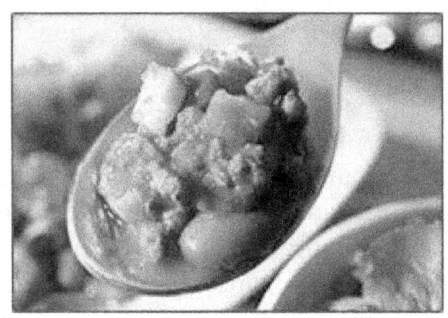

Ingredients

1 onion, yellow
1 garlic clove
1 pound beef, sirloin, ground, extra lean
1 cup tomato sauce, no-added-salt
1/8 teaspoon Worcestershire sauce
1/8 teaspoon cinnamon, ground
1 teaspoon vinegar, apple cider
4 1/2 teaspoons chili powder
1/8 teaspoon cayenne pepper, ground
1/8 teaspoon black pepper
8 ounces spaghetti, cooked
2 ounces cheddar cheese, low fat
1 cup kidney beans (cooked from dry or canned without salt)
12 olives, black
4 tablespoons green onion, chopped

Preparation:

1. Peel onion and garlic; chop onion and mince garlic.
   Brown beef, onion, and garlic in a large non-stick
   skillet over medium-high heat.
2. Place meat mixture in a large saucepan and stir in the
   tomato sauce, Worcestershire sauce, cinnamon,
   vinegar, chili powder, cayenne pepper, and black
   pepper. Simmer, uncovered, over low heat for 1 hour.

3. When meat mixture has about 20 minutes of cooking time left, bring a large saucepan of water to a boil over high heat.
4. Add pasta to boiling water and cook for 8 to 10 minutes or until al dente; drain and set aside.
5. Dividing evenly among 4 serving plates, serve meat mixture over cooked spaghetti and top with cheese, beans (drained), olives (chopped), and green onion (chopped).

Arroz con Pollo

Prep Time: 15
minutes
Total Time: 30
minutes
Serves: 4

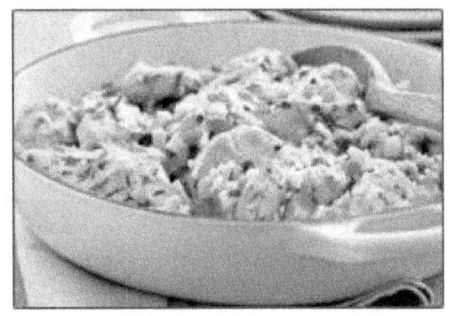

Ingredients

1 cup white rice, dry
1 1/2 cups water
3/4 cup roasted chicken breast, cubed
1/2 cup green peas
1/4 cup diced bell peppers
1/4 cup chopped onions
1 teaspoon ground cumin
1 teaspoon ground coriander

Preparation:

1. Place all ingredients into a rice cooker or covered medium saucepan and cook until done, about 25 minutes.
2. Serve hot.

Spicy Grilled Chicken and Potato Fingers

Prep Time: 15 minutes +
30 minutes of
refrigeration
Total Time: 60 minutes
Serves: 4

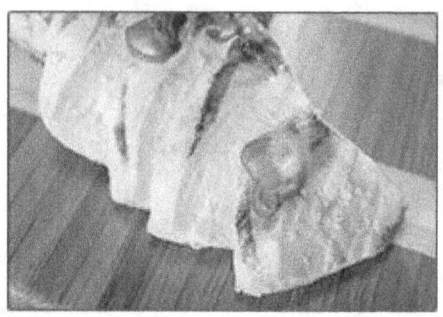

Ingredients

1 pound chicken breast, boneless/skinless, raw
2 tablespoons olive oil, extra virgin
3 tablespoons hot sauce
1/2 teaspoon cayenne pepper, ground
1/2 teaspoon black pepper
1/4 teaspoon salt
3 garlic cloves
3 baking potatoes, medium

Preparation:

1. Cut each chicken piece lengthwise into 3 strips. Place chicken in a resealable plastic bag or set in a shallow dish.
2. For marinade, in a small bowl, stir together oil, hot sauce, cayenne, black pepper, salt, and garlic (peeled and minced).
3. Pour 2 tablespoons of the marinade over the chicken; seal bag. Refrigerate for at least 30 minutes, turning bag occasionally. Cover and chill remaining marinade for basting.
4. Drain chicken, discarding marinade in bag. Preheat grill.
5. Scrub potatoes and cut each into 8 wedges. Lightly brush potatoes with some of the reserved marinade.

6. Place potatoes on the rack of an uncovered grill directly over medium coals. Grill for 15 minutes. Turn potatoes.
7. Place chicken on rack next to potatoes and grill for 9 to 12 minutes more or until chicken is no longer pink inside and potatoes are tender, turning and brushing chicken once with the reserved marinade halfway through grilling.
8. Serve immediately with grilled zucchini and red bell peppers, if desired.

Maple Pecan Scones

Prep Time: 10 minutes
Total Time: 20 minutes
Serves: 24

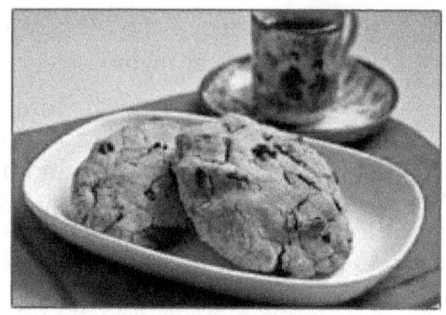

Ingredients

3 cups all purpose flour
1 cup pecans, chopped
1 ¼ tablespoons baking powder
3/4 cup butter
½ cup maple syrup
1/3 cup skim milk

Preparation:

1. Preheat oven to 375°F.
2. Combine flour, nuts, baking powder, and butter in a medium-sized mixing bowl. Mix by hand until butter is in pea-sized pieces, then add maple syrup and milk. Mix well.
3. Turn scone dough onto floured board.
4. Roll to one-inch thickness and cut in small rectangular pieces, making 2 dozen scones.
5. Place scones spread apart on a nonstick tray. Bake until firm in center and golden on edges and bottom, about 20 minutes.
6. Cool slightly and serve warm.

Blueberry Yogurt Parfait

Prep Time: 5 minutes
or less
Total Time: 5 minutes
or less
Serves: 2

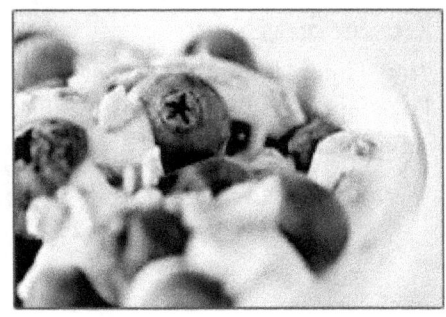

Ingredients

1 cup Greek yogurt (any fruit flavor or plain – if using plain mix with 2 teaspoons of honey)
½ cup blueberries, fresh or frozen
1 tablespoon sugar-free whipped topping, frozen
¼ cup almonds, sliced

Preparation:

1. Layer blueberries and yogurt in 2 stemmed glasses.
2. Top with whipped cream and almonds.
3. Enjoy!

To switch this up a bit you can change the flavors of yogurt and use different fruits and nuts for endless tasty variety!

Mushroom Risotto

Prep Time: 10 minutes
Total Time: 35 minutes
Serves: 4

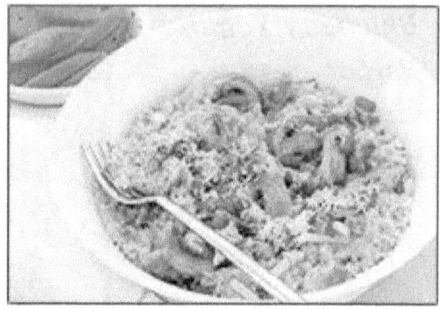

Ingredients

1 tablespoon olive oil
1 tablespoon minced garlic
2 cups mushrooms, sliced
5 cups chicken broth, heated
½ teaspoon black pepper
1 cup arborio or short-grain rice
1 teaspoon dried oregano
1 teaspoon fresh basil, chopped
¼ cup grated parmesan cheese

Preparation:

1. Heat a Dutch oven pan over medium-high heat. Add
    the olive oil and garlic and sauté until golden, about 3
    minutes.
2. Add the mushrooms and cook briefly, about 2
    minutes. Add the rice and stir well.
3. Add 1 cup of the broth, the black pepper, and the
    oregano. Bring this mixture to a boil then lower heat
    to a simmer.
4. When almost all of the liquid is absorbed, add another
    cup of broth. Stir occasionally. Continue cooking
    until all of the broth is used up, adding it in 1-cup
    increments.
5. The risotto should take about 30 minutes. Add the
    fresh basil and grated Parmesan cheese at the end.

Japanese Stir-Fry

Prep Time: 5 minutes or
less
Total Time: 10 minutes
Serves: 4

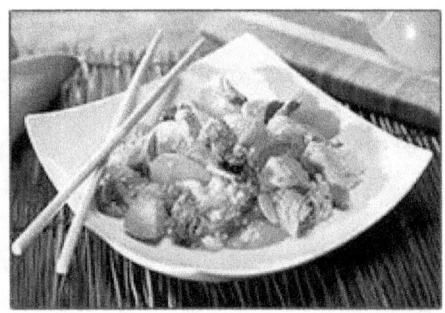

Ingredients

2 teaspoons canola oil
¾ cup snow or sugar peas
¼ cup green onions, chopped
1 cup mushrooms, sliced
1 cup broccoli florets
1 cup cabbage, shredded
1 teaspoon ground ginger
2 tablespoons light soy sauce

Preparation:

1. Heat a large, non-stick skillet over medium-high heat.
2. Add the canola oil and sauté the onions for 1 minute.
3. Add the rest of the vegetables and sauté until crisp-tender, about 3-5 minutes.
4. Season with ginger and light soy sauce.

Grilled Asparagus

Prep Time: 5 minutes
or less
Total Time: 5 minutes
or less
Serves: 4

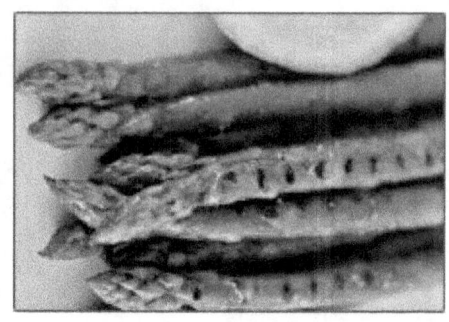

Ingredients

1 pound fresh asparagus
1 tablespoon olive oil
½ teaspoon freshly ground black pepper
Juice of one lemon (about 1 tablespoon)

Preparation:

1. Trim about 2 inches off the bottoms of the asparagus.
2. Lightly coat the spears with the oil.
3. Grill over high heat for 2 to 3 minutes, or to desired tenderness.
4. Sprinkle with black pepper and lemon juice. Serve hot.

Note – if you don't have a grill you can combine all ingredients in a shallow baking dish and roast in the oven at 350 degrees F for 15 or 20 minutes.

Useful Exercise Information

Exercising is an anathema to some people, but there are many ways to exercise that don't involve the gym or running. Walking in the park or around your neighborhood daily is a great form of exercise and burns as many calories as running does; it just takes longer to do it. If you have steps in your home or at work, walking up and down as quickly as you are able not only helps to lose weight, but can get your heart pumping!

Raising your heart rate is important for cardiac health, but if you are obese or morbidly obese this can be difficult to do. It can also be difficult to do cardiac exercises if you have injuries or other disorders. For that reason, I am only including exercises that you can do in your home or in your neighborhood. I am sure you will find them both challenging and enjoyable!

Equipment

- A chair which you can hold on to comfortably for balance. If your couch is tall enough or you are short enough, you can also use it.
- Phone book or other heavy book.
- You!

While balancing try lifting one leg up and down in a slow and controlled manner to waist height. If you can't lift your leg that high go ahead and just lift it as high as you can. Try to keep your stomach tight and your back straight as you do this in order to exercise your abdominal muscles as well. Do this eight times and then switch legs.

This exercise can be done two different ways. Try lifting your leg to the side and straight behind you to work other muscles. Though this seems like it is too easy to really work, it is a used in ballet studios across the world to strengthen muscles and it will work up a sweat!

To strengthen your arms, lift a heavy book with both hands straight in front of you until you reach shoulder height. Repeat eight times and take a break. Then lift the book directly over your head and bend your arms at the elbow directly behind your head. Do this eight times as well.

To strengthen you core, behind, and lower back, stand in front of your chair. Place your legs shoulder width apart and then bend your knees as if you were sitting, but do not sit down. Only briefly make contact with the chair before straightening up. Congratulations, you have just completed a squat! Repeat this eight times.

Finally, to strengthen your lower back lay down on your stomach. Squeeze your legs together, point your toes, and lift your arms directly in front of you about six inches above the ground. Lift your legs up six inches as well and hold this position for as long as you can. You may have noticed that you now look like Superman! By following this guide and changing your life, you probably are Superman to someone!

As you get more comfortable with exercise, you can try new methods. Try searching for exercise videos on YouTube to expand your fitness horizons. Be careful however, not to try anything too ambitious because an injury can set you back in achieving your goals.

As previously discussed, by doing easy exercises like the ones provided combined with walking one to two miles daily, you will see results in about six to eight weeks. At this point it may be good to find a fitness friend who can help you to be accountable and continue your new active lifestyle!

Conclusion

Congratulations on finishing this guide and taking control of your blood sugar! By purchasing this book and following its advice you have taken great strides towards your ultimate goal of leading a healthier and more active life. Take a moment to appreciate this significant accomplishment and to reflect on what you have learned.

First, you have learned exactly what Type II Diabetes is, how it presents, and how to treat it. Not only do you know about the western medical approach to controlling your blood sugar, but you also know about the natural remedies available. The combination of these two approaches to treatment is a powerful way to take control of your Type II Diabetes.

You also now have a completely full tool box in terms of positive coping mechanisms. By changing your thought process about eating and exercising, either on your own or with a therapist, you now have the tools you need to overcome any blood sugar issues you may have been experiencing. You are also equipped with the knowledge that you may fail, but that you can forgive yourself and move on. You also have permission to celebrate your victories when they come along. Reinforcing your good habits is essential to continuing on your lifelong journey.

With great tasting recipes, a working knowledge of the healthier areas in a grocery store, and exercises designed to help you lose weight no matter how fit (or unfit) you are, I know you can succeed in living a healthier and more active lifestyle.

Thank you again for choosing to download *The Diabetes Solution: Take Control of Your Blood Sugar & Restore Your Health Naturally.*

Christine Weil

Please leave a review and let us know what you liked about this book by going to

https://www.amazon.com/gp/css/order-history

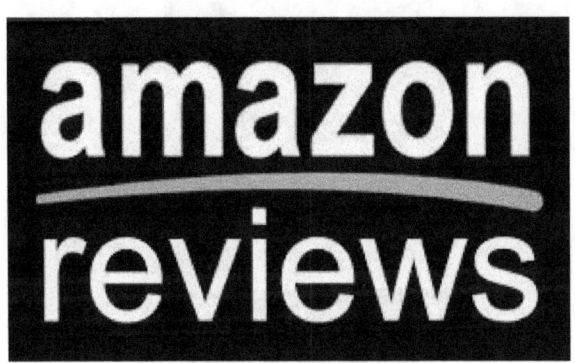

then click on Orders.

Check out the other books in the *Natural Health & Natural Cures Series*

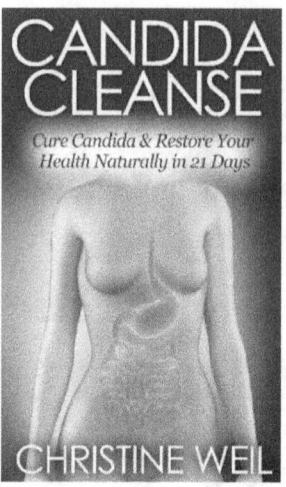

http://www.amazon.com/dp/B00IIRQH9K

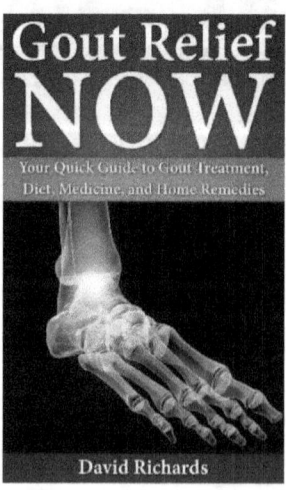

http://www.amazon.com/dp/B00HHGRBBQ

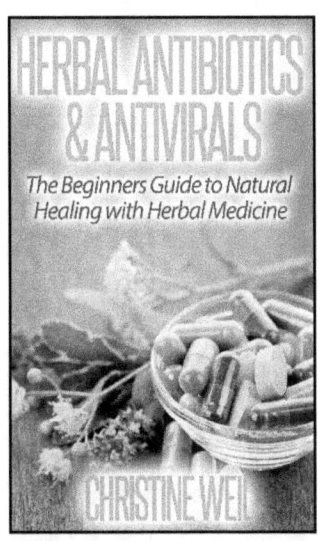

http://www.amazon.com/dp/B00J2F1QDO

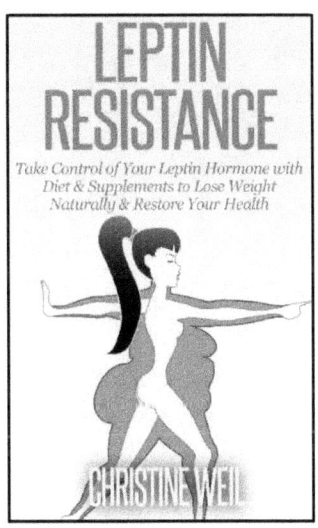

http://www.amazon.com/dp/B00J8UNBWW

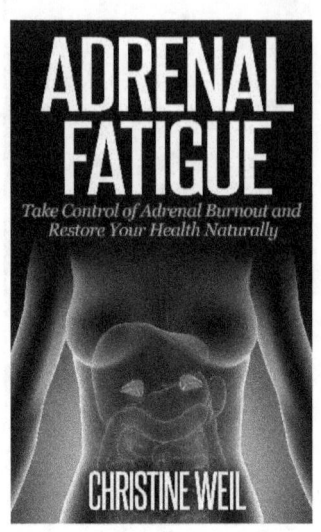

http://www.amazon.com/dp/B00J8SHS6E

www.ingramcontent.com/pod-product-compliance
Lightning Source LLC
Chambersburg PA
CBHW071636170526
45166CB00003B/1339